SAFE AND SOUND

A Healthy Body

Angela Royston

Heinemann
LIBRARY

www.heinemann.co.uk
Visit our website to find out more information about **Heinemann Library** books.

To order:

 Phone 44 (0) 1865 888066

 Send a fax to 44 (0) 1865 314091

 Visit the Heinemann Bookshop at www.heinemann.co.uk to browse our catalogue and order online.

First published in Great Britain by
Heinemann Library,
Halley Court, Jordan Hill, Oxford OX2 8EJ,
a division of Reed Educational and Professional
Publishing Ltd.
Heinemann is a registered trademark of Reed
Educational & Professional Publishing Limited.

OXFORD MELBOURNE AUCKLAND
JOHANNESBURG BLANTYRE GABORONE
IBADAN PORTSMOUTH NH (USA) CHICAGO

Designed by Celia Floyd
Illustrations by Allen Wittert, Pennant Illustration
Printed and bound in Hong Kong/China

ISBN 0 431 09140 4 (hardback)
03 02 01 00
10 9 8 7 6 5 4 3 2

ISBN 0 431 09141 2 (paperback)
03 02 01 00
10 9 8 7 6 5 4 3 2 1

British Library Cataloguing in Publication Data

Royston, Angela
 A healthy body. – (Safe and sound)
 1. Physical fitness – Juvenile literature
 I. Title
 613.7

Acknowledgements

The Publishers would like to thank the following
for permission to reproduce photographs:
AllsportUSA: S Bruty p22; Bubbles: L Thurston p4, I
West pp10, 11, 13, J Woodcock p19; J Allan Cash
Ltd: pp5, 21; Trevor Clifford: pp8, 9, 12, 14, 15, 16,
17, 20, 29; Robert Harding Picture Library: p26;
Collections: L Taylor p25; Carol Palmer: p23; Tony
Stone Images: B Ayres p28.

Cover photograph reproduced with permission of
Trevor Clifford.

Every effort has been made to contact copyright
holders of any material reproduced in this book.
Any omissions will be rectified in subsequent
printings if notice is given to the Publisher.

The Publishers would like to thank Julie Johnson,
PSHE consultant and trainer, for her comments in
the preparation of this book.

Any words appearing in the text in bold, **like this**,
are explained in the Glossary.

Contents

Healthy exercise

This girl is chasing her sister. The boys are playing in the sea. They are having fun and **exercising** their bodies.

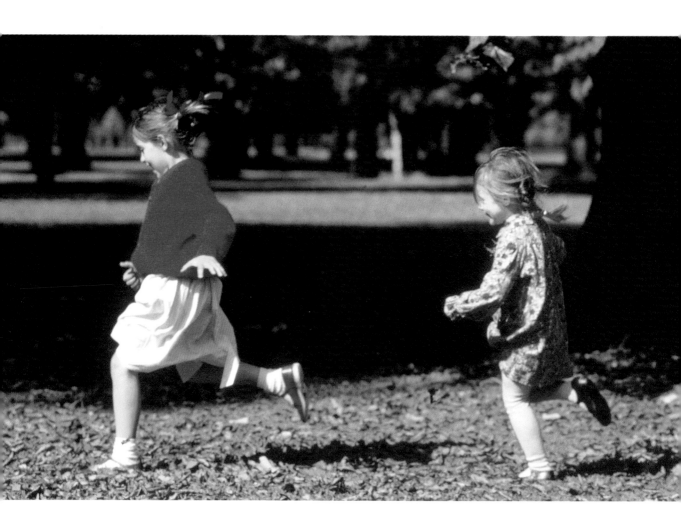

Exercise makes you fit. It keeps your **muscles** strong. It helps your **heart** and **lungs** to work well. It stops you getting too fat.

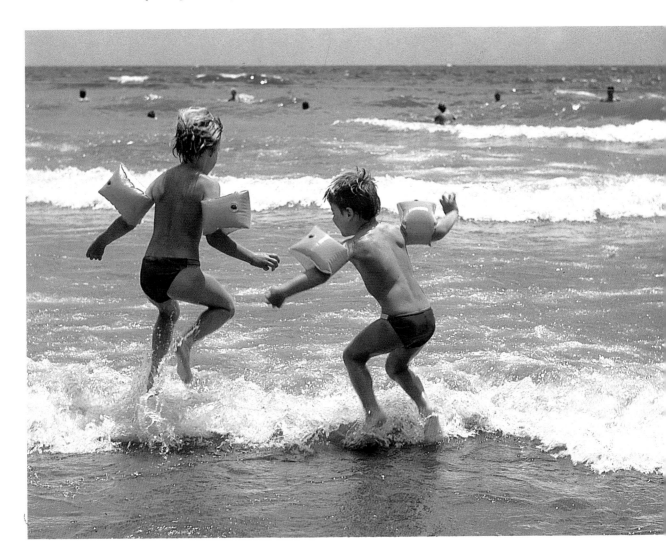

Exercise pyramid

The **exercise pyramid** shows the things you can do to keep fit. You should spend lots of time doing the kinds of things shown at the bottom of the pyramid.

You can spend less time doing the things in the middle of the pyramid. Watching television is at the top of the pyramid. It is restful, but it will not make you fit.

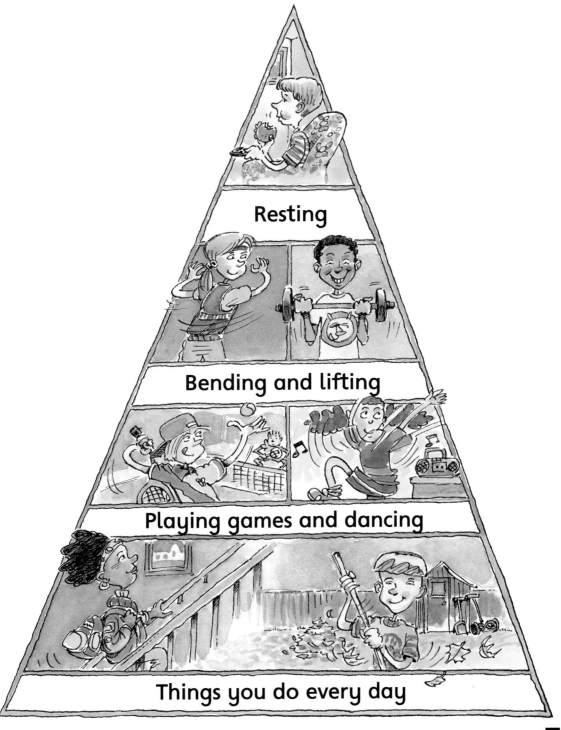

Resting

Bending and lifting

Playing games and dancing

Things you do every day

What are muscles?

Feel your arm. Can you feel the soft **muscle** and hard **bone** under your skin? The muscles are joined to the bones. They make the bones move.

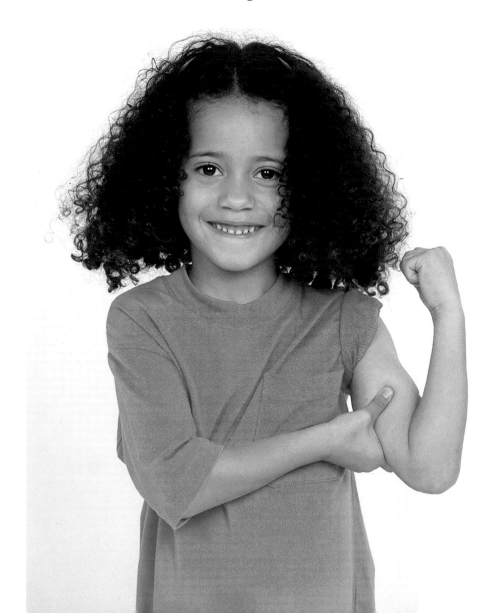

Stretch one of your legs and point your toes.
Can you feel the muscle on the back of your
leg becoming tight and hard?

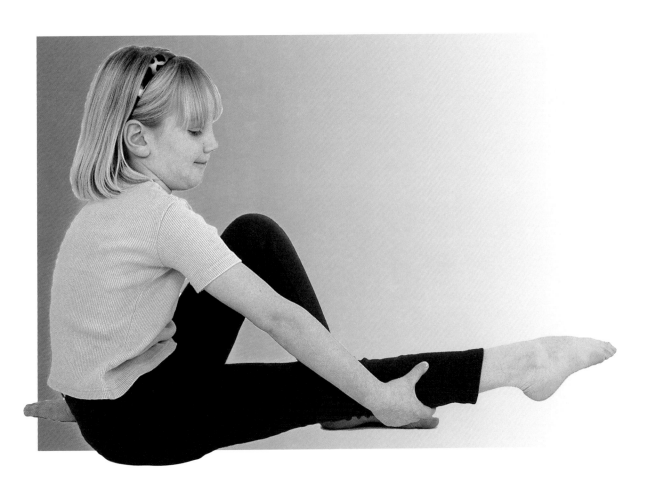

Muscle power

The more you use your **muscles**, the bigger and stronger they get. Running and kicking a ball makes the muscles in your legs stronger.

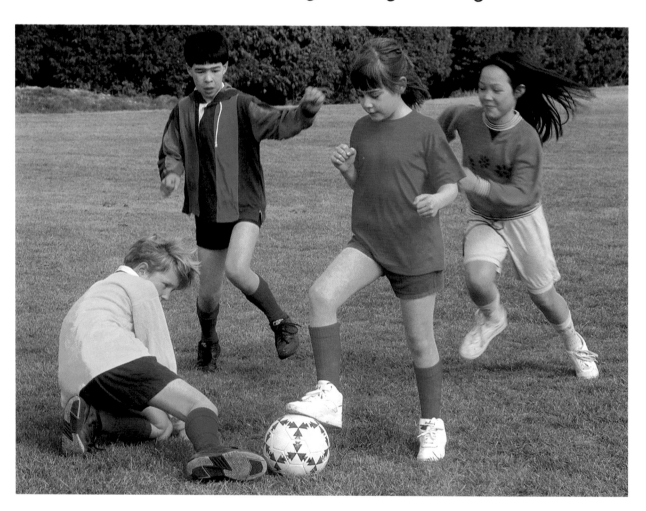

Swimming uses muscles all over your body. You move your legs, arms, back and head as you swim through the water.

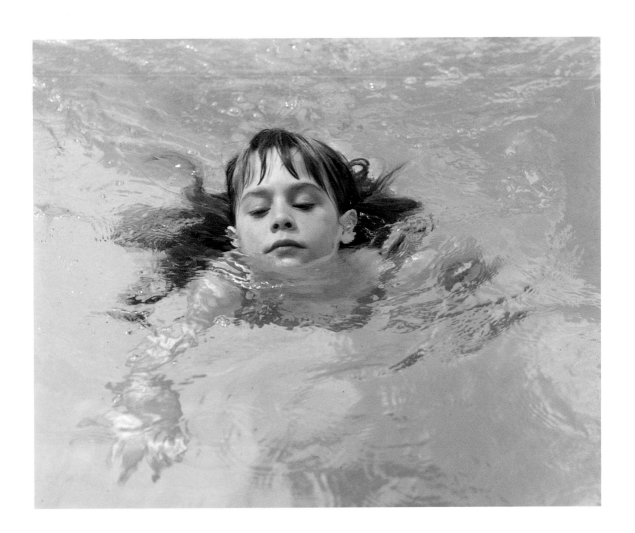

Joints

Bones cannot bend. You can only bend your body at a **joint**. A joint is where two bones meet. Which joints is this boy bending?

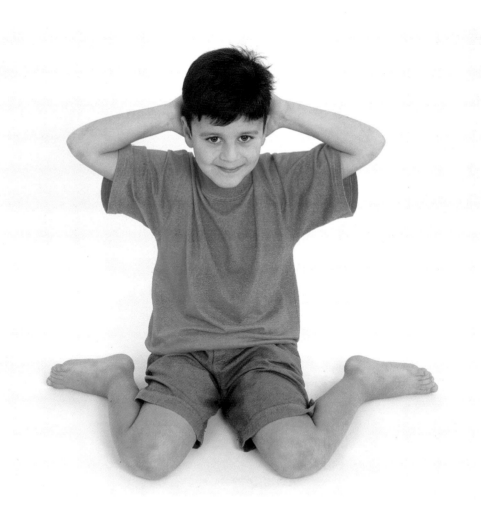

Playing on a climbing frame uses joints in your arms, hands, legs and back. It helps to keep your joints moving well.

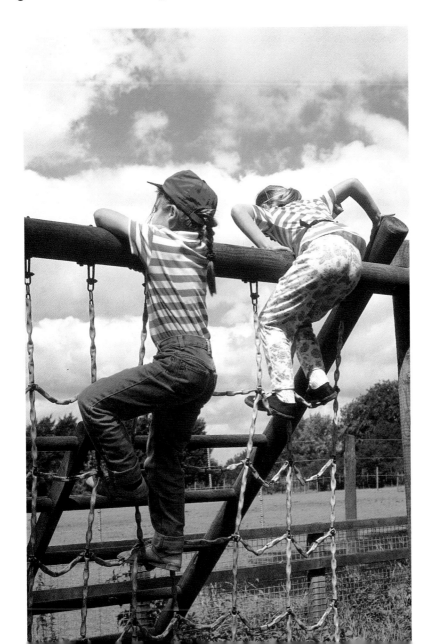

Bending and stretching

Some people can move their **joints** more than others. Can you sit cross-legged like this? You may need to practise.

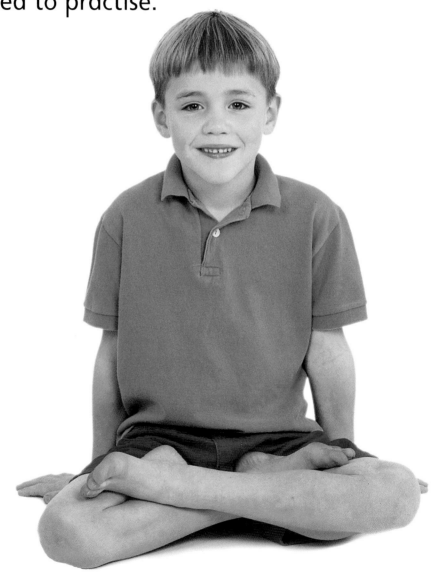

The joints in your back let you bend backwards as well as forwards. Try to make an arch shape with your back like this. Look at how this boy has placed his hands.

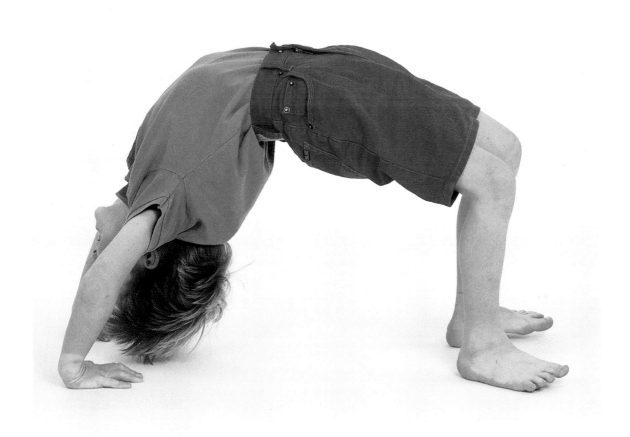

Standing and lifting

You use your **joints** and **muscles** even when you are standing still. Move your shoulders back and down to make your back straight.

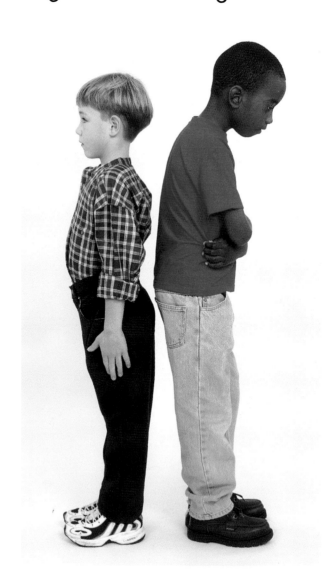

Lifting heavy things can hurt the joints in your back. Always bend your knees and keep your back straight before lifting something heavy.

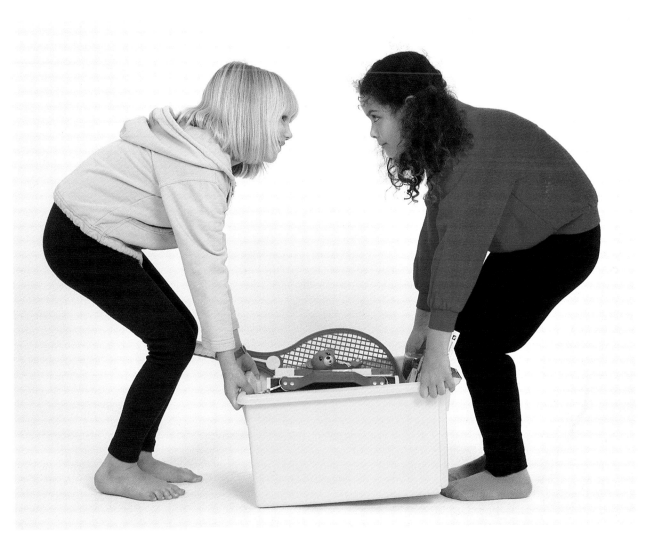

Puffing and panting

Your body needs **oxygen** which you breathe into your **lungs**. Your lungs fill with air, just like this balloon.

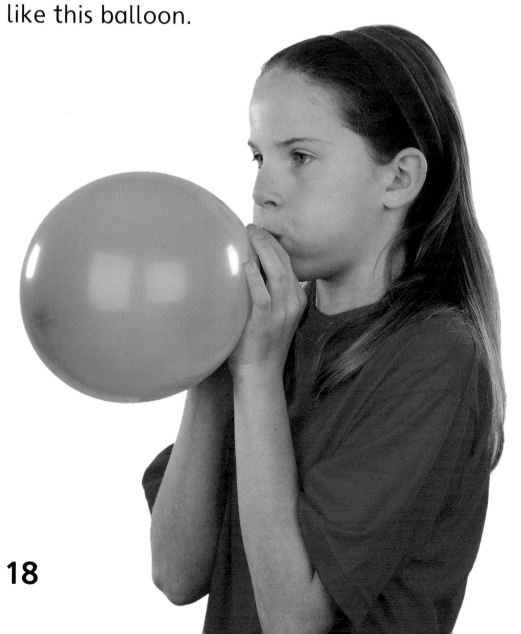

When you run you need more oxygen, so you breathe in more air. Does running hard make you puff and pant?

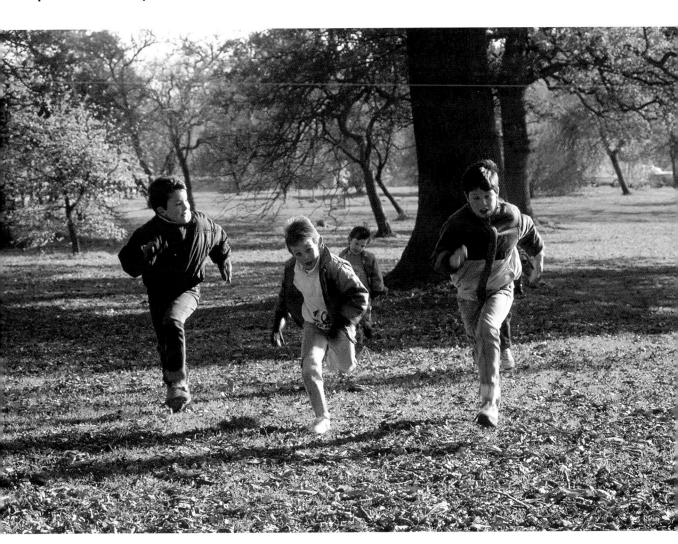

Exercising your heart

Your **heart** is a **muscle** too. Can you feel it beating in your chest? Your heart pumps **blood** around your body. Blood carries food and **oxygen**.

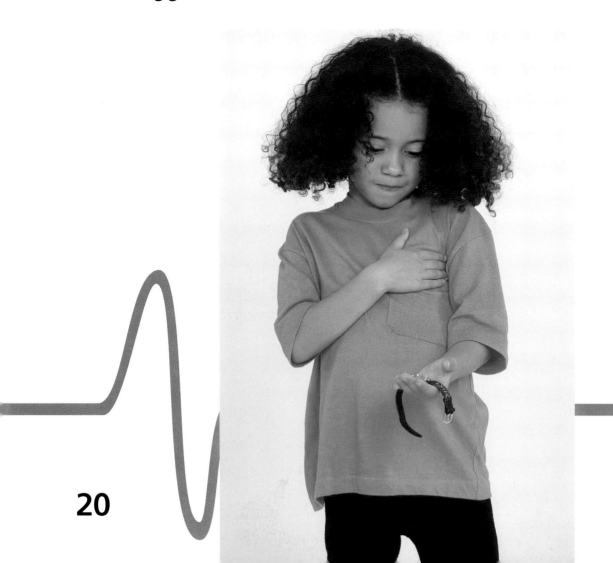

When your muscles work hard, your heart beats faster to give them more oxygen. **Exercise** makes your heart and **lungs** work better. It also makes you hot and thirsty!

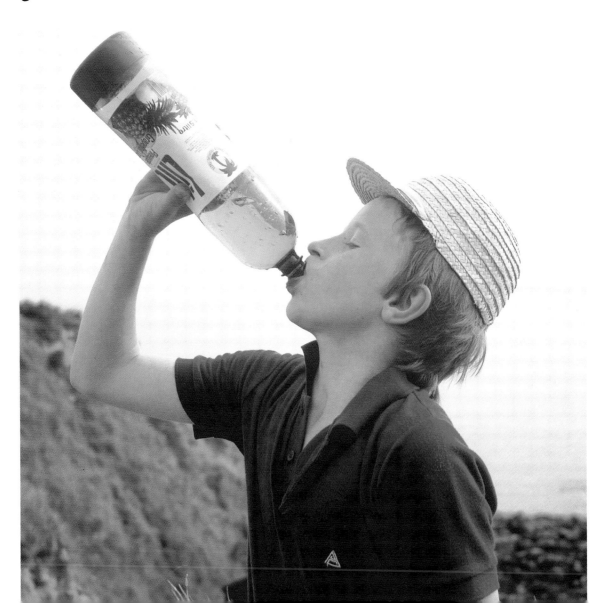

Balancing act

It is hard to balance when you first begin to skate. It takes lots of practice until your **muscles** get used to working together.

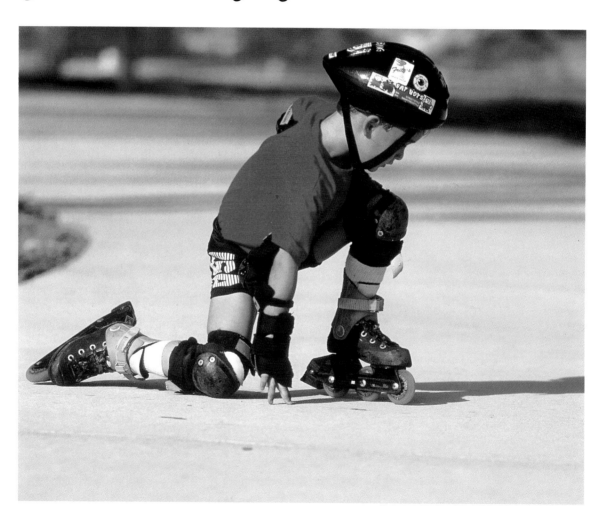

Dancing teaches you how to balance. It also helps to make your muscles stronger.

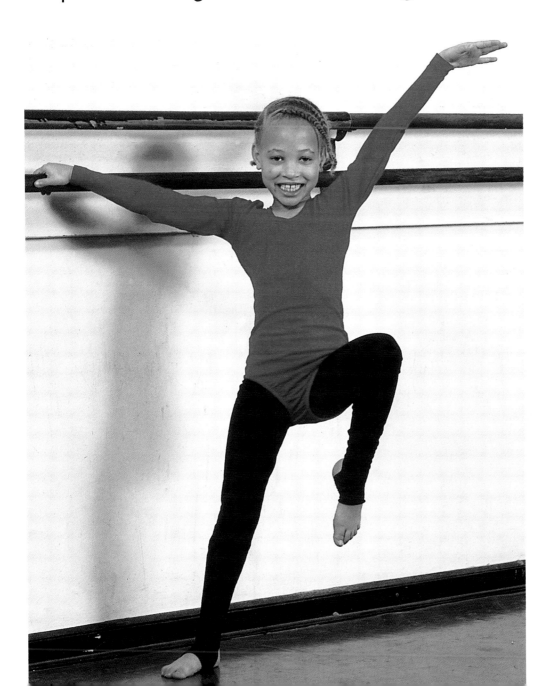

Ball play

When you throw and catch a ball you use more than just your **muscles**. Your hands and eyes work together to help you catch the ball.

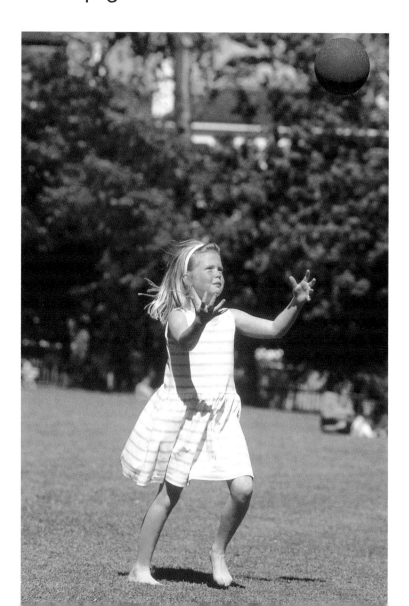

Juggling is even harder! It takes a lot of practice to **co-ordinate** your eyes and hands like this.

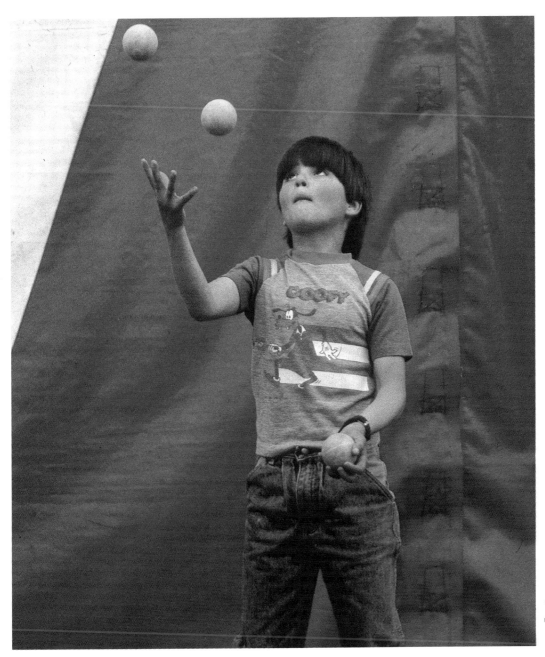

All together

Cycling uses **muscle** power, balance and **co-ordination**. A cycle ride with your family can be lots of fun.

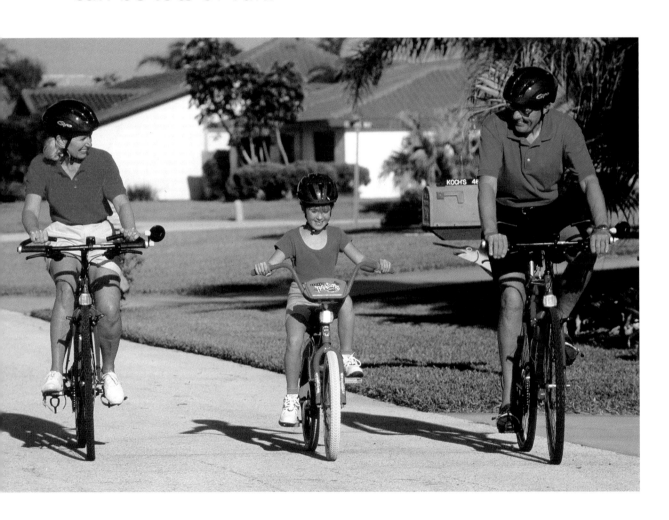

The more you **exercise**, the fitter you get. If you are fit you can exercise without getting tired.

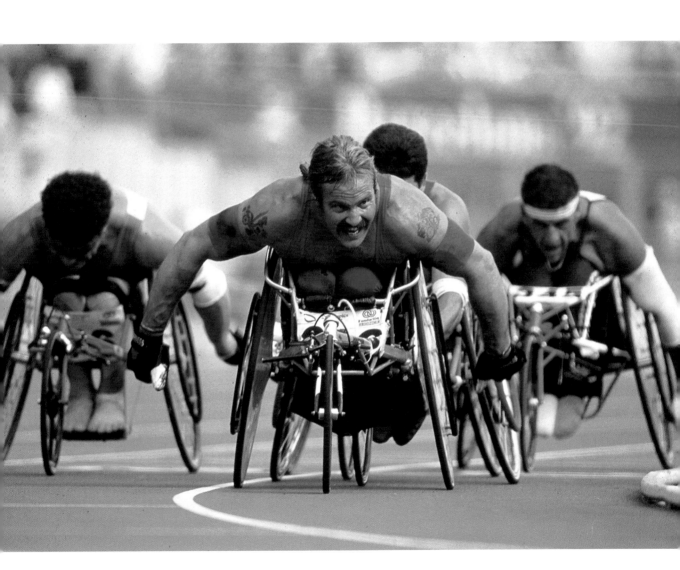

Resting and playing

To be really fit you need to **exercise** every day. Always walk to and from school if you can. It is better for your health than going by car.

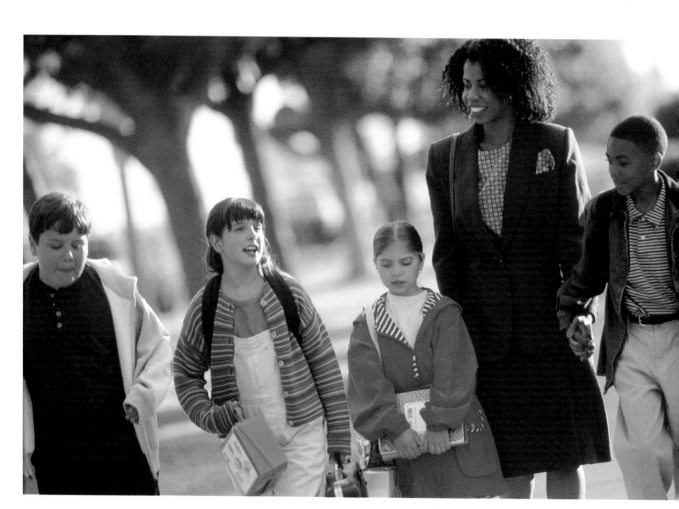

However fit you are, you need to rest sometimes. Sleep well. Your body is getting ready for another busy day!

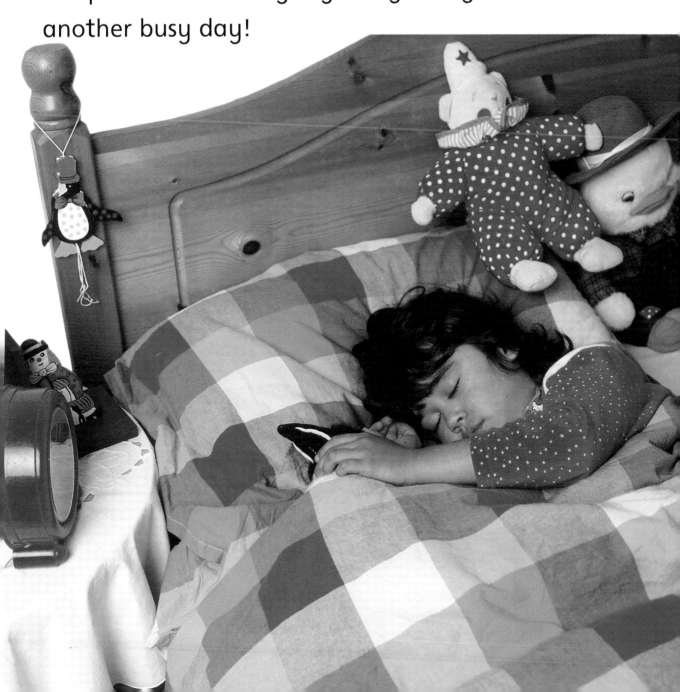

Glossary

blood   red liquid that carries food and oxygen around the body

bone   hard part of the body. Bones are joined together to give your body its shape.

co-ordinate   make different things work together

co-ordination   when different parts of the body work together to do something

exercise   something you do that uses your muscles and makes your body fitter and stronger

heart   part of the body which pumps blood around the body

joint   where two bones meet. Joints allow you to bend your arm, leg and other parts of your body.

30

lung   part of the body used for breathing

muscle   part of the body that moves the bones

oxygen   gas which makes up part of the air. All living things need oxygen to stay alive.

pyramid   object on a square base that is wide at the bottom but has a narrow point at the top

Index